Seniors
Health

Stay Fit and Healthy As You Age

RON KNESS

Sneak Peek

When you're young you have plenty of agility, and you move easily, however, as you age, well that's another story. Your muscles can become stiff, and you may find you're not as flexible as you used to be. You may feel aches and pains after simple exercise, that you never felt before. To counteract this, it's important to stay flexible so that your mobility is not impaired.

To maintain your flexibility and mobility, you need to keep active through physical activities and exercise. While aerobic and strength exercises are important, stretching is one of the best things you can do.

But there are also other areas to watch as you age, such as:
- Balance
- Posture
- Health conditions and ailments
- Hygiene and grooming

Balance
As we age, our balance is not as good as it was when we were younger. Falls from losing one's balance is the number one reason seniors break hips and other bones. And because we don't heal as fast as we used to , some lose their indepdendance and never fully regain their mobility.

Posture
Postural stoop is a common condition of many seniors. However there are things seniors can do to prevent it from happeninging. Maintaining good posture prevents other conditions of the body from happening.

Health conditions and ailments
From the heart ot headaches, health conditions and ailments seem to creep up slowly as we grow older. While all of these can't be prevented, many can be or at least their effects minimized.

Hygiene and grooming

Many seniors don't do as good as job as they should in this area. Taking care of your skin, teeth, hand, feet and nails are just as important know as they were when younger. As a matter-of-fact more important as we age.

In my new 49-page book *Seniors Health*, we cover these topics and more in an effort to keep you as young, functional and healthy as possible for as long as possible.

Published by:

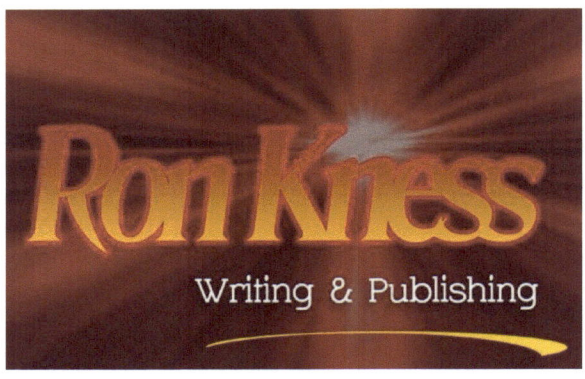

Ron Kness

San Tan Valley, AZ

United States of America

ISBN: 9781082776380

Seniors Health

Disclaimer

We hope you enjoy reading this publication, however we do suggest you read our disclaimer.

All the material written in this document is provided for informational purposes only and is general in nature.

Every person is a unique individual and what has worked for some, or even many, may not work for you. Any information perceived as advice must be considered in light of your own particular set of circumstances.

The author or person sharing this information does not assume any responsibility for the accuracy or outcome of your use of the content.

Every attempt has been made to provide well researched and up to date content at the time of writing. Now all the legalities have been taken care of, please enjoy the content.

Introduction

One of life's many cruel realities is that we don't get the rulebook or cheatsheet in advance. At every stage of our life, we can look back and say "wow, if only I'd known that beforehand", but by then it often too late.

This does not only apply to our youthful years – there are many elderly who wish that as they aged they had taken action in specific areas of their lives.

These actions could have prevented or delayed the effects that are generally related to, or attributed to, growing older. These effects, or 'conditions' invariably lead to a diminishing of the joy of experiencing life, as is experienced through reduced mobility or impairment of the senses.

At the extreme, they also cause reduced longevity.

This ebook is not a dry 'why is it so' text. Although it will help you understand why and how our bodies react as we age, it is focused on practical 'how-to' instructions and advice, to help you stay younger, longer.

Stretch to Stay Flexible and Improve Mobility

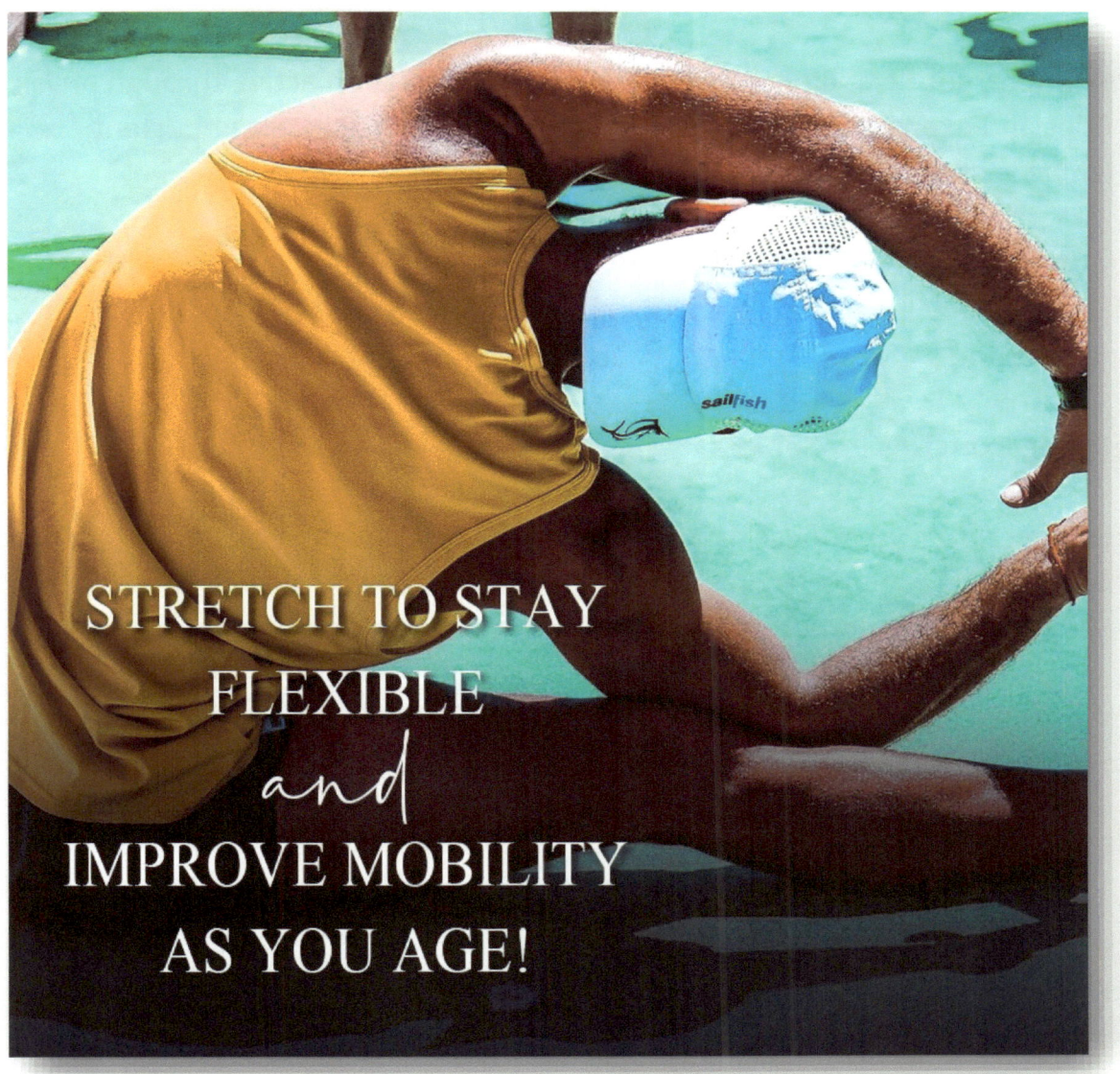

When you're young you have plenty of agility, and you move easily, however, as you age, well that's another story. Your muscles can become stiff, and you may find you're not as flexible as you used to be.

You may feel aches and pains after simple exercise, that you never felt before. To counteract this, it's important to stay flexible so that your mobility is not impaired.

To maintain your flexibility and mobility, you need to keep active through physical activities and exercise. While aerobic and strength exercises are important, stretching is one of the best things you can do.

If you stretch every day, and at least twice a day would be better, for ten minutes each time, you will be amazed at your results. You can start off small, but then develop routines that will improve your mobility even more.

Stretching Exercises for Seniors

Stretching relaxes your muscles and lubricates your joints to relieve pain and stiffness. You need to focus on your neck and spine to reverse your forward head movement, and to improve posture and balance.

Numerous neck and spine muscles are shortened or lengthened due to forward head posture. Plus, any muscle imbalance causes neck pain and back pain.

Neck Stretch

Neck stretches help improve your posture and the mobility of your neck and shoulders. You will notice the benefits from this stretch, especially when you're driving. If your neck is more flexible, you will have a better range of vision as your neck will have better rotation.

Bring your chin towards your chest and then roll your head to the right. Hold the position for 15 seconds and then do the same to the left side. Continue doing this stretch at least ten times.

Shoulder Stretch

This stretch helps with the raising, lowering, and straightening of your arms. It improves the range of motion in your shoulders and strengthens your chest muscles, which helps correct your posture. It allows you to extend the function of your shoulder ligaments, tendons, and muscles. This increases your flexibility in your shoulder joints.

Sit with your back straight and your feet firmly on the floor. Put your hands behind your head and stretch your arms so that your shoulders roll up and back. As you do push your chest out and inhale deeply while stretching. Take three deep breaths before you release your clasp, and then continue repeating the stretch.

Chest Stretch

This exercise will strengthen your chest muscles and support good posture. If you slouch, it can cause neck and back pain. This is because you tend to stick out your chin as you hunch over.

To start this stretch, extend both your arms to the sides, palms facing forward. Move your palms backward, chest out, and stretch until you feel the tension on your chest and arms.

Hip Stretch

The hip stretch increases your mobility and loosens your hip muscles for better flexibility. With your feet together on the floor, put your hands on your waist. In a clockwise direction, circle your hips five times as wide as possible. Don't move your head and shoulders while you elongate your spine and keep your stomach in. Do another five circles counterclockwise.

Back Stretch

The back stretch aligns your spine to reduce lower back pain, reduce tension on your shoulders and neck, and improve your posture. Start with your feet shoulder-width apart on the floor. Interweave your hands at chest level about 6 inches away from your chest, with your palms facing outward and your elbows pointing out.

Keep your lower body stationary and your head in line with your torso, while twisting your upper body from side to side, leading with your elbows. Try not to move your hips and keep your gaze forward. Stretch to a mild tension 10 times doing this alternately left to right. When your spine is in better alignment, you will reduce stiffness and soreness.

Hand and Finger Stretch

Hand and finger stretches make your joints strong and flexible. You can either stand or sit-down, whichever is comfortable for you. Stretch both arms forward with your palms facing outward. Pretend there's a wall in front of you, then walk your hands up until they reach above your head.

Keeping your hands above your head, wiggle your fingers for 10 seconds and then walk your hands back down.

Stretching Tips

If you have medical conditions, such as arthritis or back pain, ask your doctor if there are specific stretching exercises you should, or should not be doing. They know your history, so they can make modifications if necessary.

Do a 5 to 10-minute warm-up before stretching. You may think your stretches are a warm-up, however, start small and then stretch further. Your warm-up may include walking or gentle overhead arm circles.

Practice belly breathing by slowly inhaling and exhaling while stretching. Every deep breath fills the body with oxygen and helps improve blood circulation, which relaxes your muscles. If you hold your breath, it causes your muscles to tighten and makes any stretching exercise more difficult.

Stretch until you feel a mild tension in your muscles. Hold it for 15 to 30 seconds and don't overextend. If you feel any pain, it means you are putting too much pressure and strain into your routine, which may cause joint or muscle injury. Also, avoid bouncing, as this can damage your muscles or connective tissue.

Seniors Can Improve Their Balance with Exercises

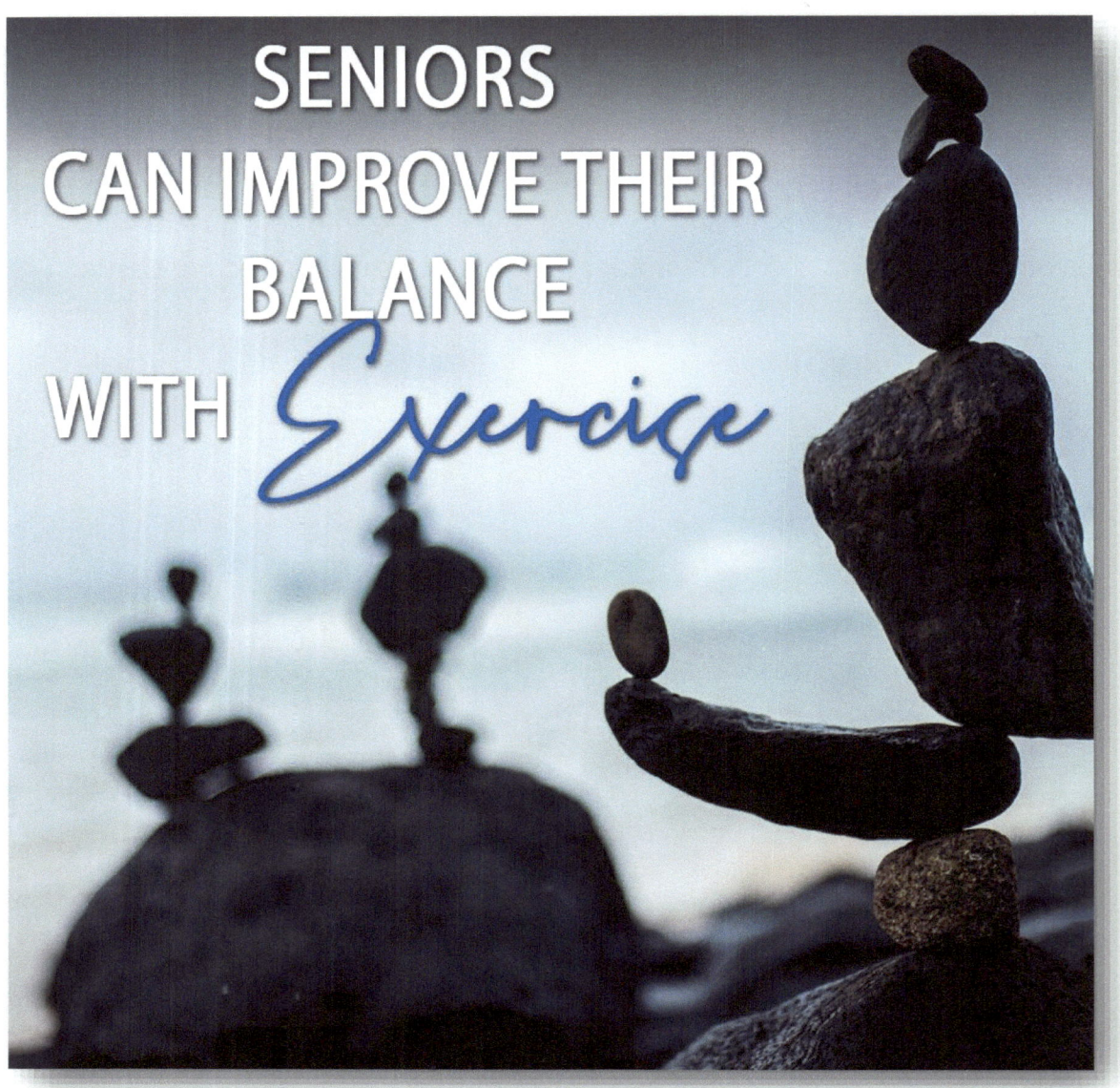

There are some obvious and some not so obvious changes in your body as you age. The not so obvious ones are things like muscles that have lost their strength and mass and flexibility, and your reaction time diminishes.

You may begin to move slower, take shorter steps when walking, and be extra careful so you don't fall. Falling is something many seniors are afraid of. Getting off balance and taking a fall can mean a fracture or broken hip.

Physical factors that can create instability and throw you off balance include:

- Carrying excess weight
- Inactivity and poor mobility
- Eating an unhealthy diet, causing deficiencies of essential vitamins and minerals
- Health conditions and medications.

Here are some tips to keep you on your feet:

- Maintain a healthy weight
- Build your diet based on your nutritional requirements
- Get plenty of quality sleep
- Drink plenty of water
- Stretch every day.

Last but not least, exercise, exercise, exercise! You might be worried about the type and length of your exercise routines, so please consult your doctor first, especially if you have a previous or present medical condition. If you do have a medical condition, don't think you shouldn't exercise, it's vital for health, and to maintain your balance and mobility.

Exercise and physical activities can improve not only your balance but many illnesses, as exercise is part of many disease management programs. Therefore, keep moving to strengthen your body.

Exercises for Improving Balance

Here are some recommended exercises for you to improve your balance and coordination:

Heel to Toe Walk

This is a simple exercise which helps keep your legs and back strong and stable. Start in an upright position, both your feet close together and firmly on the floor. Place your right foot in front of your left so they are aligned with your right heel in front of your left toes. Move your foot in such a way that you're putting the weight on your heel.

You can repeat the process with your left and alternate making the steps with both of your feet until you make 20 steps. To have a bit of fun, imagine walking like a model, or walking on a tight rope. Keep one foot in front of the other, heel to toe, heel to toe, and allow your hips to swing from side to side to exert a little mild pressure on your spine.

Toe Lifts or Calf Raises

This exercise builds the muscles in your calves, legs, and thighs and strengthens the joints of your knees and toes. Stand in front of a bench top or counter, or a sturdy chair and put your hands on it for support. Don't lean forward. Raise up on your toes as far as you can go then lower yourself slowly. Repeat the process 20 times.

Side Leg Raise

Side leg raises strengthen your hip muscles and joints and corrects your posture. It strengthens the groin muscles too. Stand and take your position behind a counter or a sturdy chair for support. Place your feet slightly apart and keep your back straight.

Slowly raise one leg out to the side, your toes pointing forward. Keep your other leg slightly bent at the knee, so you don't put undue pressure on the knee. Alternate with the other leg 10 to 15 times and repeat the process.

Important to Remember

While doing these exercises, it's important to remember to breathe deeply. Deep breathing delivers oxygen to your muscles and helps increase your lung capacity. Plus, you make your workout and post-workout recovery faster.

Resistance Training or Weight Training Benefits

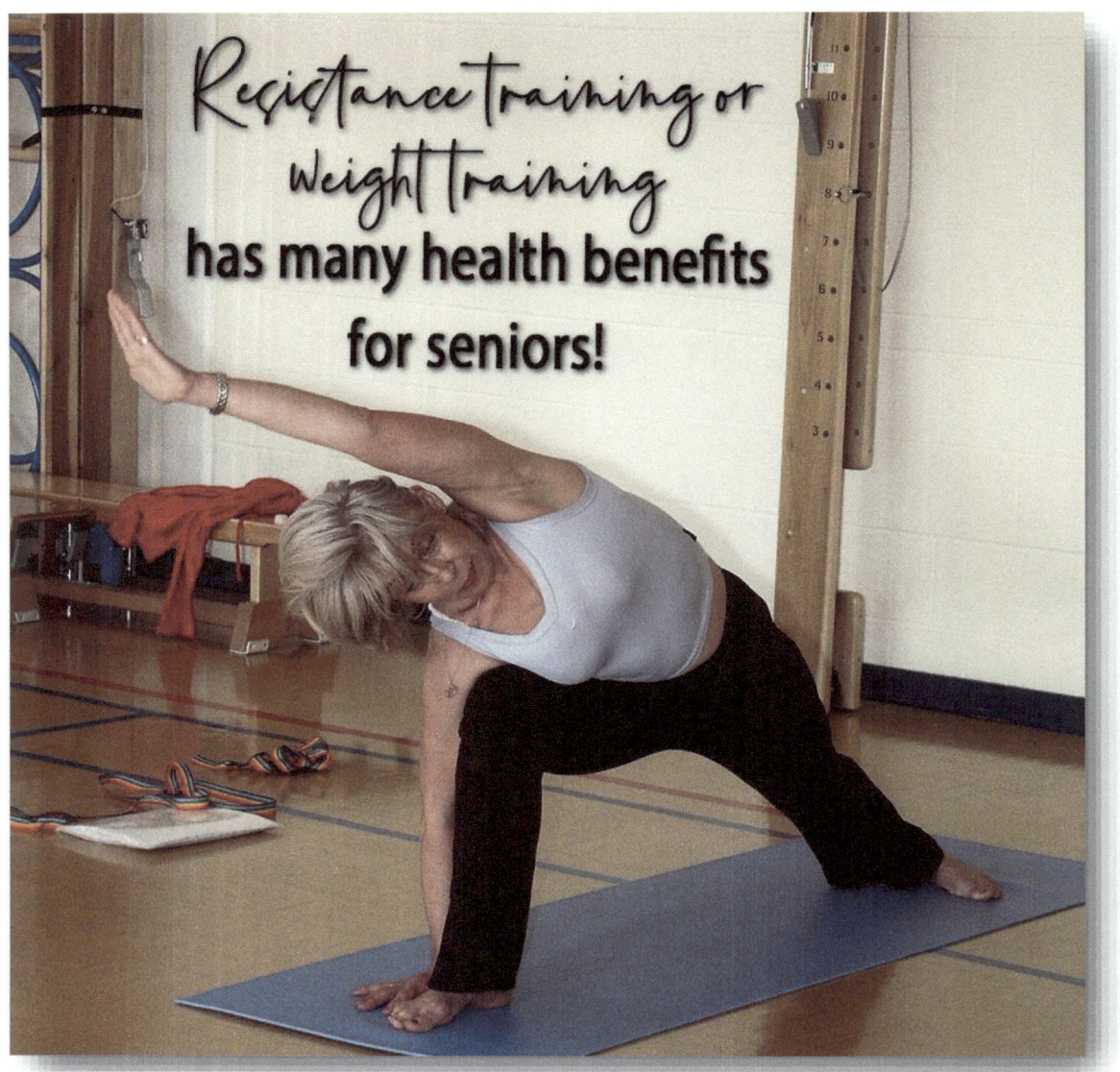

Are you over 50 and considering hitting the gym to lift a few weights? If so, good for you! It's never too late to start regardless of your age. It's actually very beneficial if you do.

There are many physical health benefits if you start resistance training or weight training, and there are mental health benefits too. For one, if you join a gym, you'll have the opportunity to socialize!

Advantages of Training with Resistance or Weights

Here are just a few of the advantages of exercising with weights, or even your own body weight.

Improves ligament flexibility, muscle strength, and muscle mass.

Your muscles and ligaments are made up of different proteins. The predominant one is collagen, which provides structure and strength. There is also elastin which allows your muscles to snap back into shape after being stretched (for ligaments) or contracted (for muscles).

By using weights or resistance techniques, you work your tissues against a force which gradually makes them stronger. The ligaments extend to their full length, which helps increase your range in motion. The flexibility gained in your joints improves your balance, which helps against falls and improves your mobility. The last thing you want as you age is to lose your ability to move freely.

Regular resistance training makes your muscles contract to increase strength and muscle mass. If you have strong muscles, instead of atrophied, weak muscles, your skeleton can stand strong, which means improved bone and joint health.

Remember that muscle strength is more important than muscle mass, so focus on the intensity and progression of your exercising. When you increase the repetitions and the amount of weight, you will be increasing the demand on your muscles. This helps gain strength, size, endurance, and increase muscle functionality.

Another benefit is that if you are eating a healthy diet, your body will begin to burn stored body fat for energy as you work out. Therefore, you will lose fat in the process and become a lean machine!

It is recommended that you do weight resistance exercises at least twice a week if you're a beginner in order to achieve maximum benefits. Since you have likely lost muscle mass as you have aged, because of reduced physical activity, you will need to work hard to regain it.

Resistance training slows or reverses the process of aging. It can slow or even stop the decline in muscle mass, bone density, and strength. That statement alone is worth getting started right now!

Manage blood pressure, blood sugar, and blood cholesterol levels.

Studies show that when your body mass index or BMI - the indicator of body fat - increases, there's a corresponding increase in your blood pressure. Elevated blood pressure levels are a risk factor for cardiovascular disease and stroke.

Another problem with an increase in weight and age is that you may develop higher triglyceride, cholesterol, and blood sugar levels. They increase your risk of heart disease, stroke, diabetes, and kidney problems. If you have any of these conditions or are extremely unfit or overweight, consult your doctor before undergoing resistance training.

However! You can benefit from weight training if you have these conditions.

Both moderate-intensity dynamic resistance training and low-intensity isometric resistance training induce a significant decrease in blood pressure levels. Plus, there are favorable effects, in the reduction of triglyceride levels. Training can also prevent and control type 2 diabetes by increasing insulin sensitivity, which leads to lower blood sugar levels.

Good for your cognitive functions and awareness.

Cognitive decline is a major health concern among seniors, specifically dementia and Alzheimer's disease.

If you lead an active life throughout your youth and senior years, you may prevent these degenerative diseases, improve your memory, enhance your thinking skills, and stimulate your brain cells to grow. Your mind will stay alert and healthy.

If you couple your resistance training with aerobic exercises such as swimming, jogging or walking, it can increase the size of your hippocampus which is responsible for learning and verbal memory.

Help reduce pain and stress.

Resistance training is helpful if you have arthritis or spinal osteoporosis, so don't go thinking you can't do weights! It increases bone density and improves the muscles surrounding the afflicted area. This helps reduce pain and maintain your coordination and agility. After a while, you may find yourself climbing the stairs with ease, whereas once it was painful and almost a non-event.

Another benefit after exercise is you may notice you feel good. You may notice you are in a better mood and have a happier disposition. When you do resistance training, your brain releases endorphins. These hormones have an analgesic effect, minimizing discomfort during your workout, so you feel good. Plus, one of the hormones, dopamine, is your 'happy hormone' so you feel more upbeat.

Therefore, you relieve stress and pain, which is good not only for your body but for your mind as well. Weight training or resistance training has so many benefits as you age. What a great way to maintain your youthful body and general well-being.

Seniors Emotional Health Can Improve with Exercise

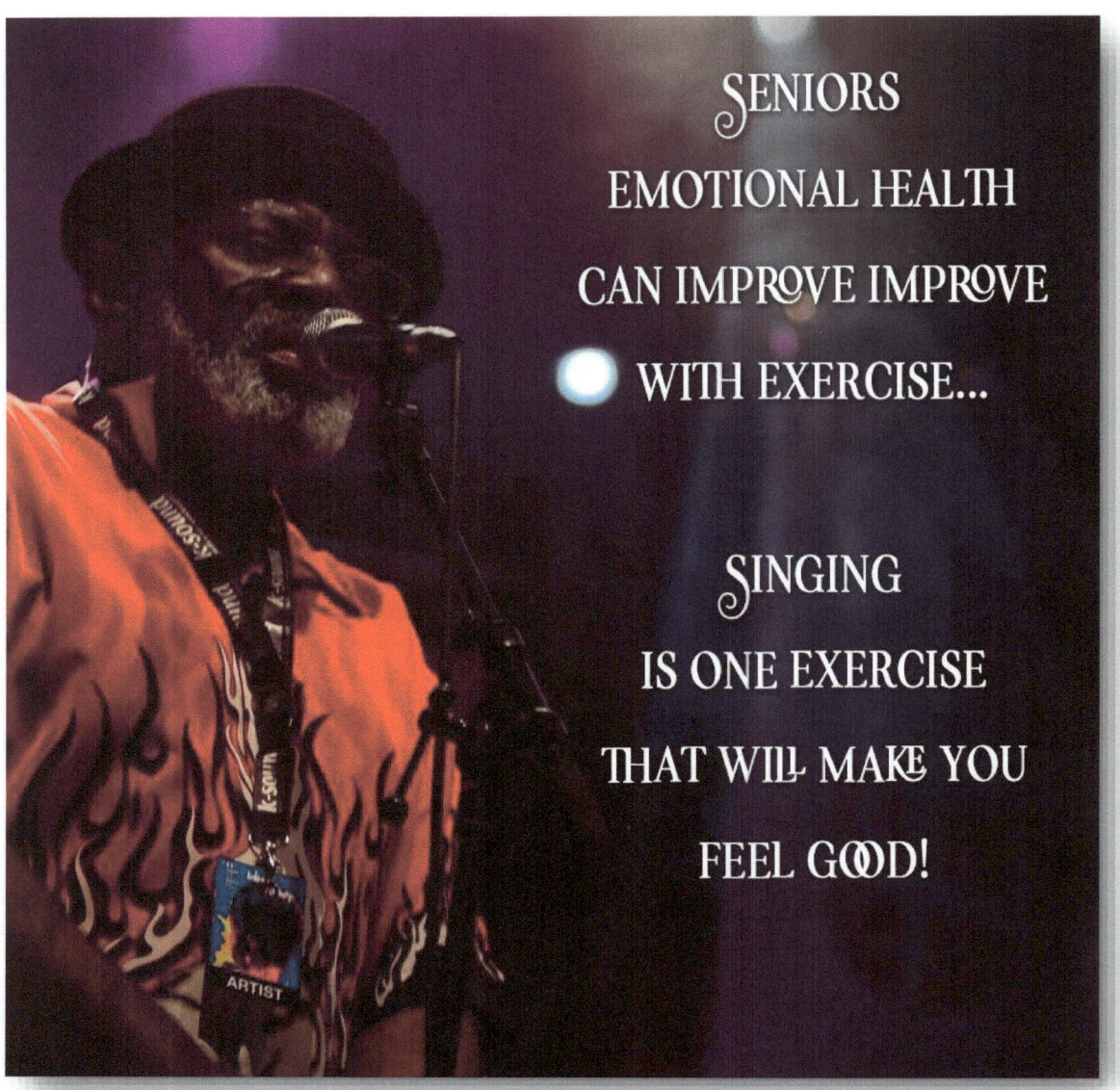

Aging effects not only our physical appearance, which can be a major concern for some people, but more importantly, there can be invisible changes in our mental and emotional health.

For example, degenerative diseases that limit mobility and coordination can result in being isolated from family and friends, which can cause stress and loneliness.

These seniors are a vulnerable group, and it's a major concern as to what can be done to improve their emotional health.

One way to do this is with exercise. Exercise is a great prescription for improving mental health and has been shown to improve mental health conditions in seniors.

There is a range of very beneficial exercise types, such as aerobic, resistance training, and stretching exercises.

Benefits of Exercise to Improve Emotional health

Here are just a few of the benefits that exercise can do for your emotional health.

Keeps you independent.

Exercise boosts emotional wellbeing. If you can remain independent and perform your daily tasks, this will keep your self-esteem and self-confidence more intact. If you can't perform simple tasks, it can make you feel hopeless and dependent.

Being elderly and being able to 'do your own thing' can give you a great sense of satisfaction, knowing you are still in control of your life and are still able to manage your daily affairs.

Having independence enhances the quality of your life. You can make your own choices or decisions. You can make simple decisions such as what to eat, what to wear and where to go. People who can't make these simple decisions have a harder time emotionally as they battle with their own sense of purpose and quality of life.

Increases social interaction.

Joining groups, whether it be fitness groups or hobby groups, can widen your social interactions. You meet new friends who share the same passion and interests. You get the feeling of belonging from your support group, which contributes to your happiness and contentment.

Within your family circle, you will have greater energy and stamina to play with your grandchildren, and to laugh at their antics. Laughter alone has many health benefits, so don't underestimate the benefits of a good old belly laugh!

If you a person who laughs often, here's how you benefit:

- Lowers your blood pressure and reduces the risk of stroke.
- Produces 'happy hormones' to relieve stress.
- Increases immune cells and antibodies, so you develop disease resistance.
- Gives your heart a cardio workout.
- Exercises your stomach muscles because they expand and contract when you laugh. (Have you ever held your stomach after laughing so hard because your stomach muscles hurt? Know that it's good for you!)
- Promotes your general wellbeing, both physically and emotionally.

Improves mood.

When you exercise, you feel happy and exude a more happy, positive disposition. You sleep better at night and feel good about life. You have the energy to do the things that you love, and you have a sharp mind. You feel younger than your chronological age.

What's Stopping You from Exercising?

You might think you're not well enough to exercise. It has been proven that exercise also improves the symptoms of degenerative diseases. There's nothing to lose but a lot to gain. You only need to develop a positive mindset about performing physical activities.

If you have a health condition, consult the professionals that can help you, such as physiatrists or physical therapists. Physiatrists are specialists who treat conditions of the nerves, muscles, and bones that affect movement. Physical therapists can help if you have health problems or injuries in your muscles, bones, or nerves.

It is harder to be happy and uplifted when in pain, or when mobility is limited due to inactivity. There's far less reason to be sad or temperamental if you feel good about yourself and life in general.

When you're active, you have much less time to linger on disruptive thoughts of 'what-if' and 'maybes.' Your physical activities help you to be mindful and keep your thoughts away from those that contribute to stress or anxiety.

Choose an exercise that you love to do. Do you love to sing? That's still an exercise! Singing makes your diaphragm strong and improves general circulation.

It produces a feeling of elation and pleasure from the release of endorphins. Singing also releases oxytocin, a hormone that alleviates stress and anxiety.

Keep Your Back Straight and Prevent Postural Stoop

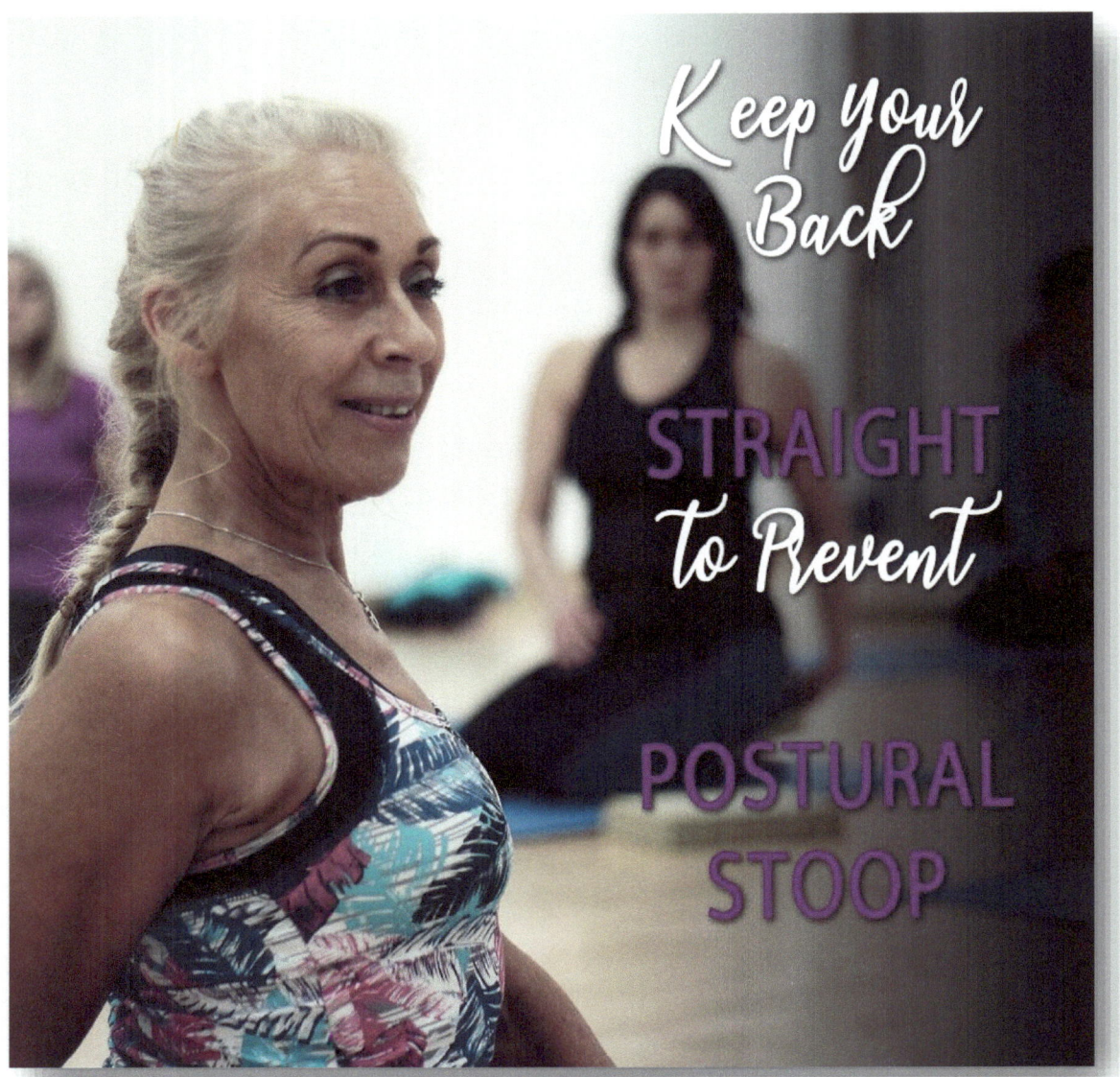

A humped back or a hunched back is something that afflicts some seniors. It's a condition where the spine bends and the back begins to stoop. You may think this is just a part of getting old.

However, physical changes which result from disease and lifestyle choices are not considered part of the normal aging process.

What Causes a Postural Stoop?

Quite often, it occurs from a vertebral fracture due to bone density loss. This is a medical condition known as osteoporosis. It often results from a lack of calcium, magnesium and vitamin D, and inevitable changes in the hormones. These lead to the weakening of the bones, which become brittle and fragile.

Osteoporosis is preventable and to a degree, reversible. Damaged discs and fractures can certainly cause damage to the spine and cause the back to stoop, but if you want to try and keep your posture and back as straight as you can as you age, here are a few tips to help you.

Keep an Active, Healthy Lifestyle

Exercises are extremely important. They will strengthen your body and help you maintain strong bones, muscles, and joints. Include weight-bearing exercises. These are activities that make you move against gravity without overstressing your bones, muscles, and joints.

Walking, dancing, and climbing the stairs are some of the weight bearing exercises you can try. Swimming is another great exercise as it strengthens your bones and muscles to improve posture and flexibility.

Another group of exercises you can do are those that strengthen your 'core.' Core-strengthening exercises build strong core muscles that help stabilize the spine and the lower back to make you stand tall.

There are exercise programs that focus on strengthening your core muscles, such as Yoga or Pilates.

Along with exercise, you need to look after your health by not smoking, or drinking excessively. You may be wondering how this can affect your posture. Smoking increases the risk and severity of osteoporosis and subsequent risk of bone fracture. It interferes with the absorption of calcium and vitamin D, which are essential for healthy bones.

Excessive alcohol consumption can also damage your bones, which affects your posture. Alcohol, like smoking, interferes with the absorption of calcium and vitamin D. Good bone health is one of the many reasons to not smoke, and to minimize alcohol consumption.

Eat a Rich Calcium, Magnesium and Vitamin D Diet

Calcium is very important for building strong bones, and magnesium is required for calcium absorption. The recommended daily intake of calcium for women aged 50 and below is 1,000 milligrams. For women above 50, they need 1,200 milligrams of calcium every day.

There are many calcium supplements available. However, natural food sources are best. Good sources of calcium include milk, cheese, and dairy products, salmon, almonds, tofu, and dark-green leafy vegetables.

Although calcium is the major mineral in bone composition, recent research strongly indicates that most people are not lacking in calcium intake. No matter how much calcium is ingested, if the body is lacking in other essential nutrients, primarily vitamin D and magnesium, the calcium is not absorbed as it should be and is excreted.

D3 is the type of vitamin D needed for calcium absorption. Women up to the age of 70 need 600 IU while 800 IU is recommended for women 70 and older. The best source of vitamin D is for you to soak up the morning sun, on bare skin, such as forearms. You can also source vitamin D from eggs, saltwater fish and liver.

Avoid Prolonged Sitting

Prolonged sitting is bad for your posture as it can cause you to round your shoulders and make your back stoop. Therefore, be conscious of how you sit. Sit with your spine straight and your shoulders back.

Keep your knees at a 90° angle and your feet flat on the floor. Your weight must be distributed equally on both hips.

Don't lean your weight on one side and change your position every 30 minutes or get up and walk around. If you have been sitting for more than an hour, you should definitely get up and get moving. This makes your muscles stretch, facilitates blood circulation and encourages bone growth.

While you are sitting, even if sitting correctly, your body is not being stressed by gravity as it needs to, to trigger bone formation. Even if you can't walk, or engage in another exercise, standing is so much better than sitting for long periods.

Prolonged sitting compromises your posture bigtime!

If you are spending a lot of your time sitting at a computer, avoid leaning forward as this places strain on your neck and back muscles. Using an ergonomic chair is recommended to help you maintain a correct posture while sitting.

Heart Healthy Habits for Seniors

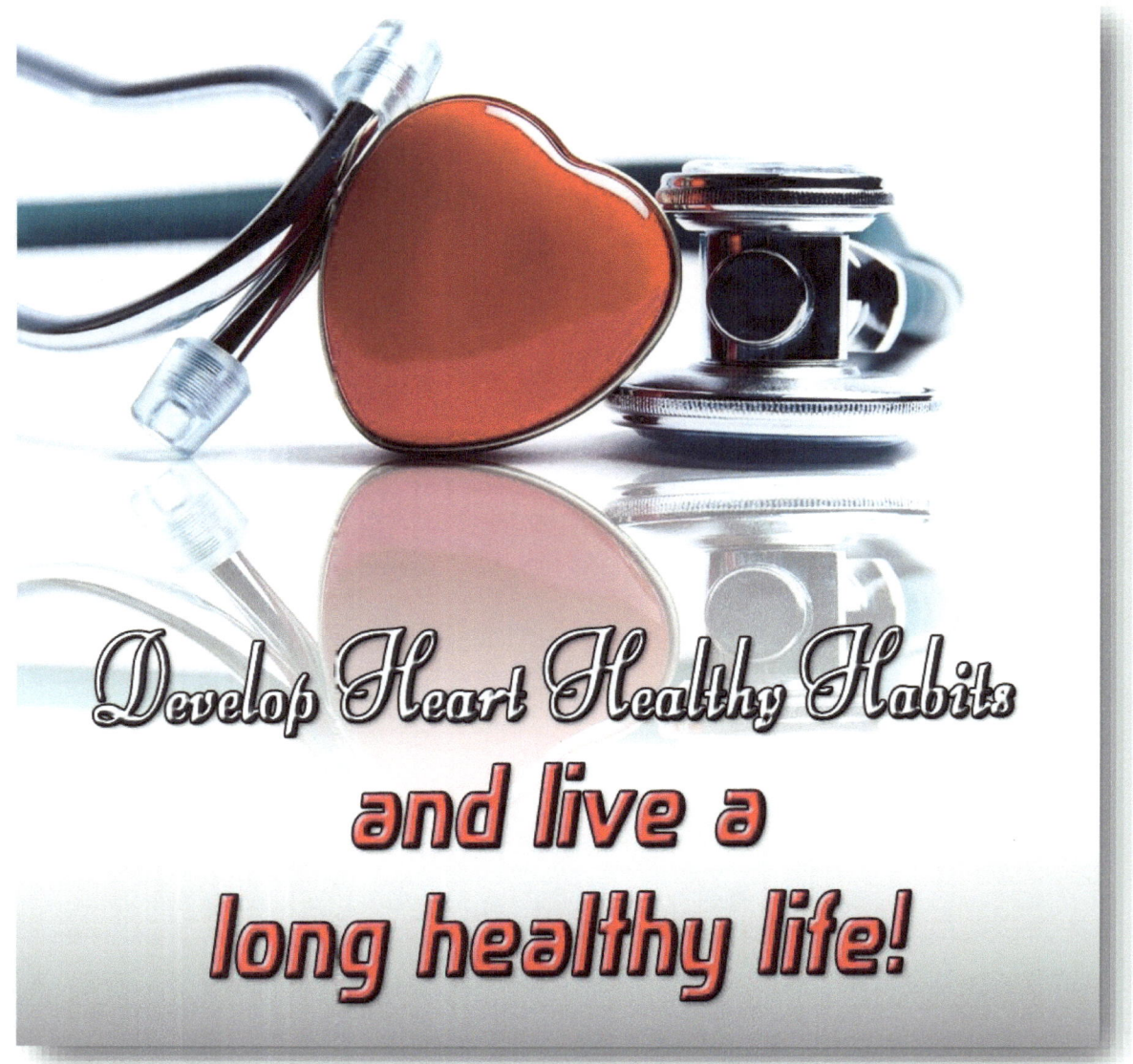

If you have taken good care of your heart when you were younger, your heart is probably in good shape now. However, even if you were a little careless about your heart health in you~ youth, you certainly can, and should, start now. It's never too late to start.

If you have heart-healthy habits, you will improve the quality of your life and live longer. Heart disease is the leading cause of death in the United States.

Most of these deaths are seniors over the age of 65. This may sound alarming; however, heart disease can mostly be prevented. Despite your years, you can get started in making this muscle a strong one! Here are some tips to help you get started.

Exercise Every Single Day

Regular exercise helps you to stay active, keeps you physically fit and makes your heart stronger. It is recommended that you exercise 30 minutes every day.

You don't need to sign up for a gym membership as there are plenty of heart-healthy exercises you can do either in the comfort of your own home, or in your street. Taking a simple walk is one of the best exercises you can do for your heart health. Here are the benefits of taking a walk.

- Reduces the risk of heart disease and stroke
- Increases cardiovascular and pulmonary fitness
- Improves other medical conditions that might lead to a heart attack, such as hypertension (high blood pressure), high cholesterol, and diabetes.

You can also start a 'physical activity hobby' such as dancing. If you are having fun, you are also reducing your stress levels. Doing so will also help lower your resting heart rate and blood pressure levels.

Eat a Heart-Healthy Diet

Your diet has a direct impact on your heart health. Eating the right foods can help prevent heart attack and other heart diseases.

Eat food rich in antioxidants and enzymes that protect the cells from damage brought about by free radicals. Examples of antioxidants are beta carotene, lycopene, or anthocyanin. One of the most powerful is hydroxytyrosol which is found in olive oil.

To boost your antioxidant intake, types of food to eat include olives, berries, avocado, beets, red cabbage, tomatoes, and green leafy vegetables.

Omega-3 fatty acids are excellent for heart health. They help lower blood pressure and cholesterol levels. Omega 3-rich foods include fatty fish such as salmon and sardines. You can also get omega 3 from chia seeds, and some nuts, such as walnuts, almonds, macadamia nuts, and hazelnuts.

Whole oats have a high amount of fiber, which can help lower cholesterol. They are also rich in antioxidants including avenanthramides that may lower blood pressure levels.

Avenanthramides increase the production of nitric oxide, a molecule that helps dilate blood vessels and facilitate better blood flow and circulation.

Socialize

You may have experienced feelings of depression, loneliness, stress, anxiety or hopelessness which are all risk factors for coronary heart disease and stroke. Therefore, it's important to socialize and connect with people.

You can socialize by joining community groups or charities, or simply spend more time with friends and family. Just don't become isolated. Social connections alleviate negative feelings and reduce the risk of heart disease and hypertension.

A happy you makes a healthy heart.

Headaches in the Senior Years

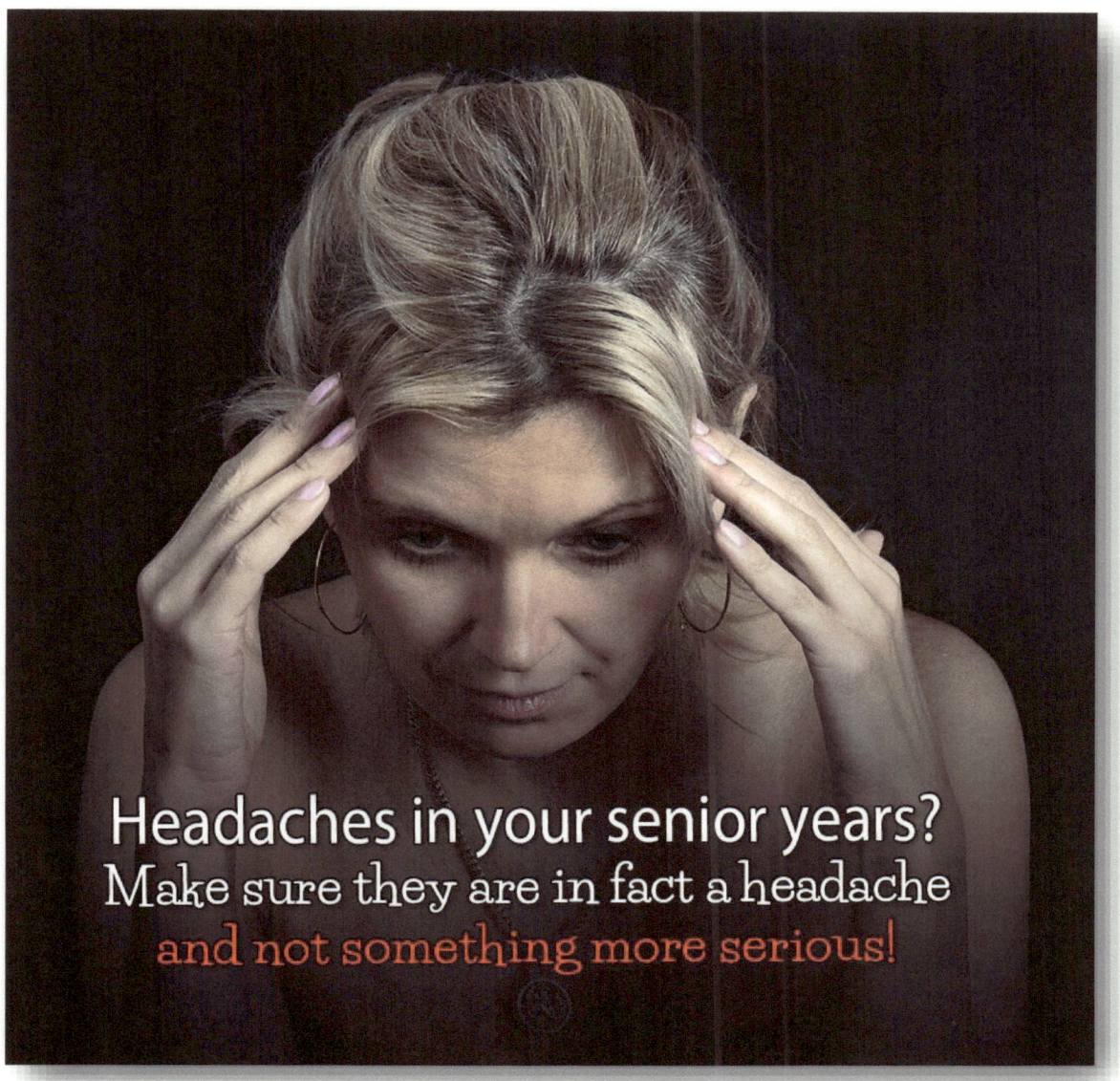

Headaches in your senior years?
Make sure they are in fact a headache
and not something more serious!

More often than not, migraine sufferers find that as they get towards their retirement years, the incidence of migraine attacks decrease.

Because headaches are generally less prevalent in seniors, if you do start experiencing an increase in headaches in your senior years, you should take them seriously and have them checked by your doctor.

You won't have headache pain unless there is a reason. If they are more regular, you should take a visit to see your doctor just to make sure there is no underlying problem.

It may be just a headache due to stress, or the food you ate last night, but there is no need to take any chances. It is far better to visit your doctor and be told to go home and take a rest than to have a stroke or worse.

Here are a few of the common headaches seniors may experience. If you have never suffered from headaches in your youth, (lucky you if you didn't), the following explanations will help you determine if you are suffering from a particular type of headache or not.

Migraine Headaches

Migraine headaches usually come with warning symptoms or what is known as an aura. You may feel pain or tingling on one side of your head. Then you may feel a throbbing or pulsing pain, become extremely sensitive to light and noise, followed by weakness, nausea and/or vomiting.

As a senior you may develop a milder type of migraine that can cause neck pain rather than headache pain. It can be caused by allergies, light, stress, and foods. If you sense anything more than a 'migraine aura', then another problem may be responsible, and you need to see your doctor immediately.

Tension Headaches

Tension headaches are a common type of headache that even people over 65 years of age may endure. Its occurrence may decrease with age. However, they can become prevalent later in life. Your muscles contract in your head and neck causing pressure and tension across your forehead.

A variety of foods can cause tension headaches such as MSG, chocolate, aged cheeses, and smoked fish. The muscles contracting can also be a response to a head injury or stress.

Massaging your head is great for relieving a tension headache. A massage on your neck and shoulders can release the tight muscles. You can even give yourself a massage by gently rubbing your fingers on the painful areas. Try a little Bowen therapy on yourself and feel the difference. It can feel much better very quickly.

Cluster Headaches

Cluster headaches are seasonal in nature because they appear at the same time of the year, every year. You may feel a series of short, extremely painful headaches, that may last from 20 minutes to 3 hours, and that continue on for weeks or months, once or twice a day.

Or you may feel as if you have one big never-ending headache that lasts for months with no relief in sight.

Due to the nature of a cluster headache, you may mistake it for an allergy or stress. The cause of cluster headaches is unknown and there is no cure. The pain can feel excruciating, but they are not life-threatening, although they can affect the quality of your life because they are the most debilitating of all.

Neck Pain in Your Senior Years

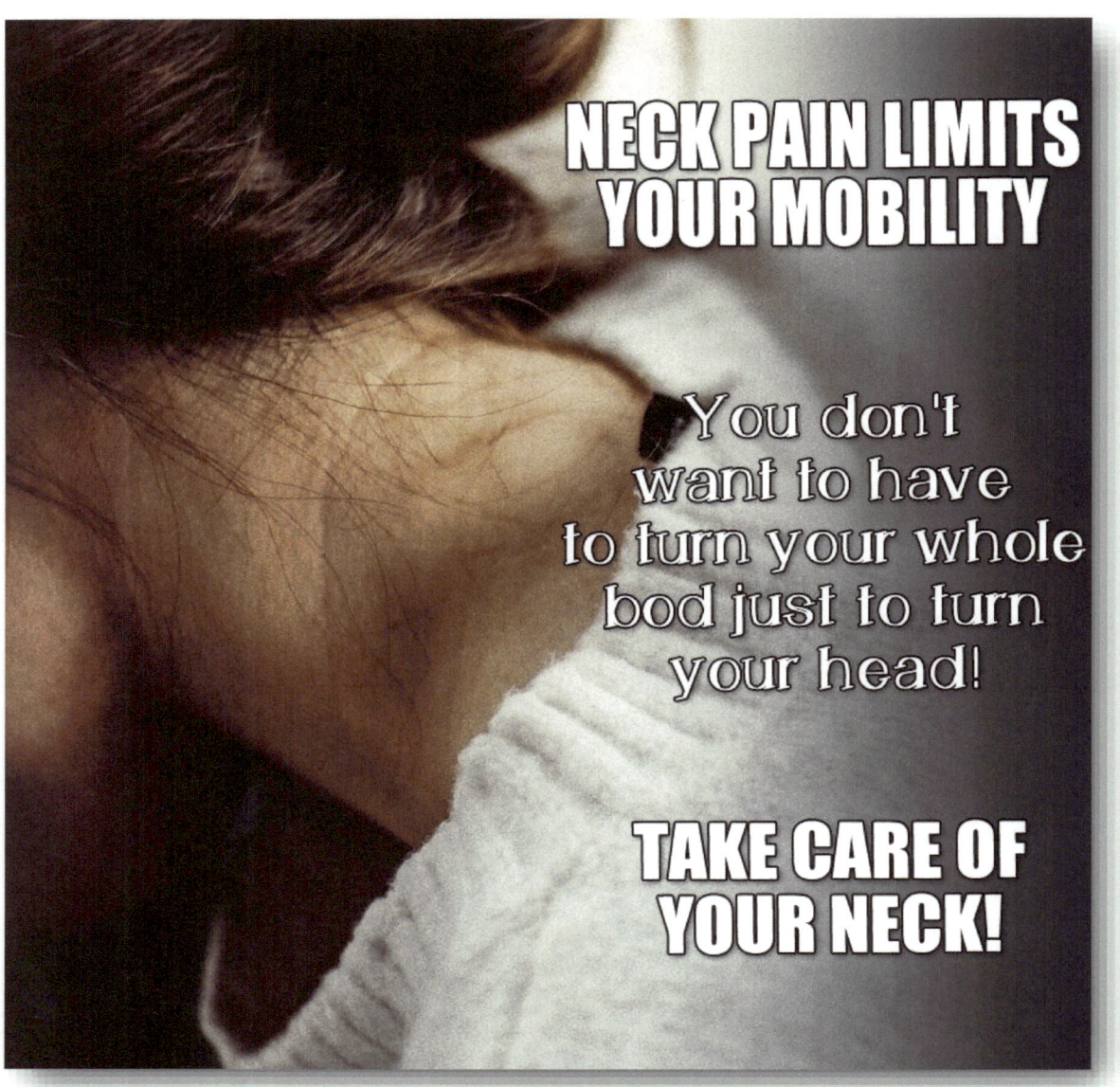

Neck pain does not start overnight. As you age, you become more susceptible to degenerative diseases that can cause lower back pain and neck pain, such as spinal osteoarthritis and degenerative disc disease.

If you have one of these medical conditions, activities in your everyday life can aggravate the pain. You might be sleeping with your neck in an awkward position, or you may have over-extended your neck muscles.

You might have unknowingly injured or strained your neck. Turning your head side to side repeatedly, holding in an unnatural position for too long, or quickly turning your head can cause pain the next day.

Here are a few tips to help with neck pain.

Cold and Heat Treatments

Place an ice pack on the area for a maximum of 20 minutes, at 30-minute intervals. After the cold application, you can then switch to applying heat, with the use of a heating pad or a hot towel compress.

The temperature should be comfortable enough not to burn. Applying heat increases the blood flow, which brings proteins, oxygen, and other nutrients to help in the healing process.

Stretching

Stretch your neck muscles gently by moving your head from side to side slowly. You can also do shoulder roll exercises to release muscle tension. Roll your shoulders clockwise then counterclockwise to increase the strength of your upper back and neck to increase flexibility.

While you are stretching and exercising, make sure you breathe deeply. Deep breathing has an analgesic effect, as well as a 'de-stressing' effect on the mind, which allows muscles to relax and pain to diminish.

Stay Hydrated

Drink plenty of water to keep you hydrated. This will help nourish your discs. These are the spongy structures that lie between the vertebrae in your spine.

If you keep them hydrated, they will be plumper and provide you with a neck and back that will be able to act as a shock absorber.

The discs are mostly water, about 70% when you reach the age of 70, compared to 85% in children, and this decreases with age. Proper hydration makes them more pliable and healthy.

Watch Your Posture

Good posture lessens the pressure in your neck, whether you're sleeping, standing, or sitting. Sleep on your side or back with an orthopedic pillow that will give you the right support and elevation to avoid strain on your neck.

When you're sitting or standing, don't stoop! If your head is in a neutral position or normal head posture, as opposed to a head poked forward, the stress on your neck is minimized.

This is because the weight of your head is balanced on your spine. If it's poked forward, it becomes a much heavier weight. You can check if your head is in the right position - your ears will be aligned with your shoulders.

Neck pain limits your mobility. You don't want to have to turn your whole body just to turn your head. Take care of your neck as you can't replace it!

Back Pain and Stiffness

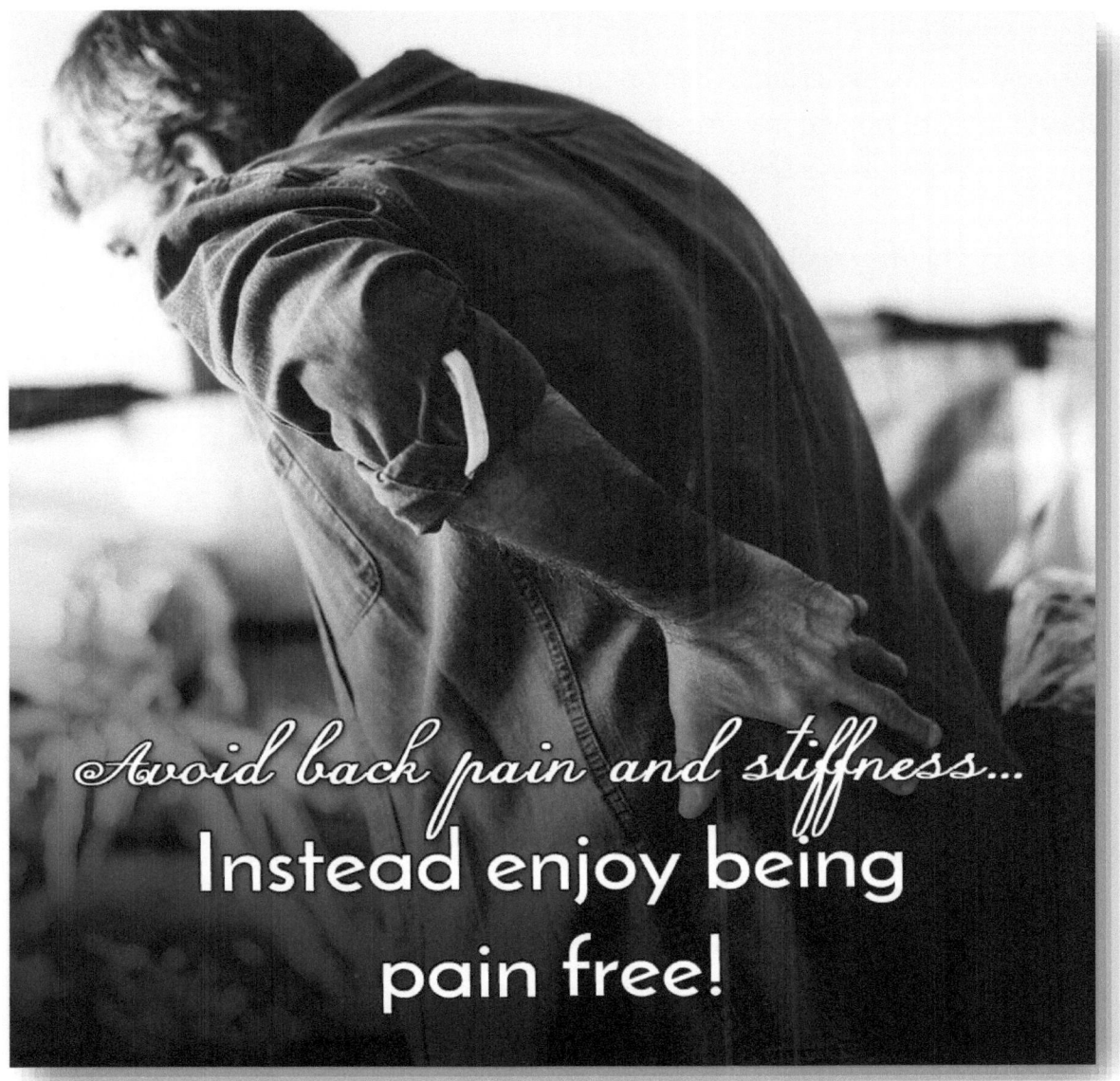

Avoid back pain and stiffness... Instead enjoy being pain free!

Do you suffer from back pain and stiffness, especially in the morning? Perhaps you feel great through the day, maybe a little stiff, but by morning you feel as stiff as a board. It may be difficult to even roll out of bed.

There are many reasons why feeling stiff and achy can occur in your senior years. Your sleeping position, your pillows, or your bed could certainly be a culprit.

However, even mild physical activities you do the day before can exert pressure and subject your spine to discomfort and pain in the morning, not to mention feeling stiffness.

Of course, you may experience back pain and stiffness if you have a health condition such as spinal osteoarthritis which is the degeneration of your joints in the spine. It's a disease associated with aging and develops gradually over time.

Steps to Stay Healthy and Pain-Free

There are things you can do to keep your spine healthy, minimize your pain and stiffness, and maintain your movement and flexibility. Here are a few tips you can do starting right now.

Choose A Diet That Promotes Wellness

There are anti-inflammatory foods you can add to your diet to reduce pain and stiffness. These include green leafy vegetables, almonds and walnuts, fatty fish, and berries.

More importantly, there are also foods to avoid, which helps prevent inflammation. They include:
- Processed meats, such as sausages, bacon and ham.
- Processed snack foods, such as potato chips and crackers.
- Artificial trans fats – margarine and certain vegetable oils.
- Refined carbohydrates - bread, pasta, flour, white rice.
- Sugar and sugary foods - cookies, candy, cakes, pastries, sugary drinks.
- Excessive alcohol consumption.

Strengthen Your Core

You need to do stretches and exercise daily to strengthen your muscles. You can't stand straight or bend easily if your body is losing muscle tone and core strength.

Your posture is affected by the strength of your core, a lack of which can cause lower back pain and stiffness.

Done properly, these same stretches and exercises also reverse the shortening of connective tissues, such as tendons. As we age it is normal, but not not ideal, to reduce our range of movement, such as length of stride, reach, twisting and turning, etc.

Then we do have to extend ourselves, we experience pain and discomfort. Regular (daily) stetching and exercising will go a long way towards overcoming this.

Warm up before you start exercising. Warm-ups increase the blood flow to your muscles and prepares your body for your workout. This reduces post-workout muscle soreness and stiffness.

Don't Place Undue Pressure on Your Spine

When you lift something, lift it the right way! This will help avoid muscle, joint, and disc injuries. Always remember to bend at the hips not the back. When carrying heavy items, keep your chest forward and your arms close to your body.

Avoid carrying anything at arm's length.

When lifting, work through one plane of movement at a time – that is, don't lift and twist at the same time. Lift, then rotate to the needed position to place the item, then lower. Keep the movements separate.

Treat Strain and Sprain Injuries Carefully

Injuries cannot be totally avoided. Treat them properly by following the RICE - rest, ice, compression, and elevation method. As soon as possible, use an ice pack over a sore muscle to lower blood flow to the injured area.

This will reduce the inflammation that causes pain. As a rule, cold therapy is only effective in the first 24 to 72 hours of an injury.

Manage Stress

Your golden years should be as stress-free as possible. Stress causes physical pain and problems. It's not just mental anguish that stress provides. If you find you are stressing more than you should be, find out what is causing your distress and do something to fix it.

Your back pain and stiffness felt in the mornings could be coming from stress the day before! Your tension can cause tense muscles. Look for ways to relax.

Before going to bed do what you enjoy. Listen to music, read a book, take a relaxing bath. Do whatever it takes to relax your muscles, and get a good night's sleep!

Hygiene and Grooming Tips for Seniors

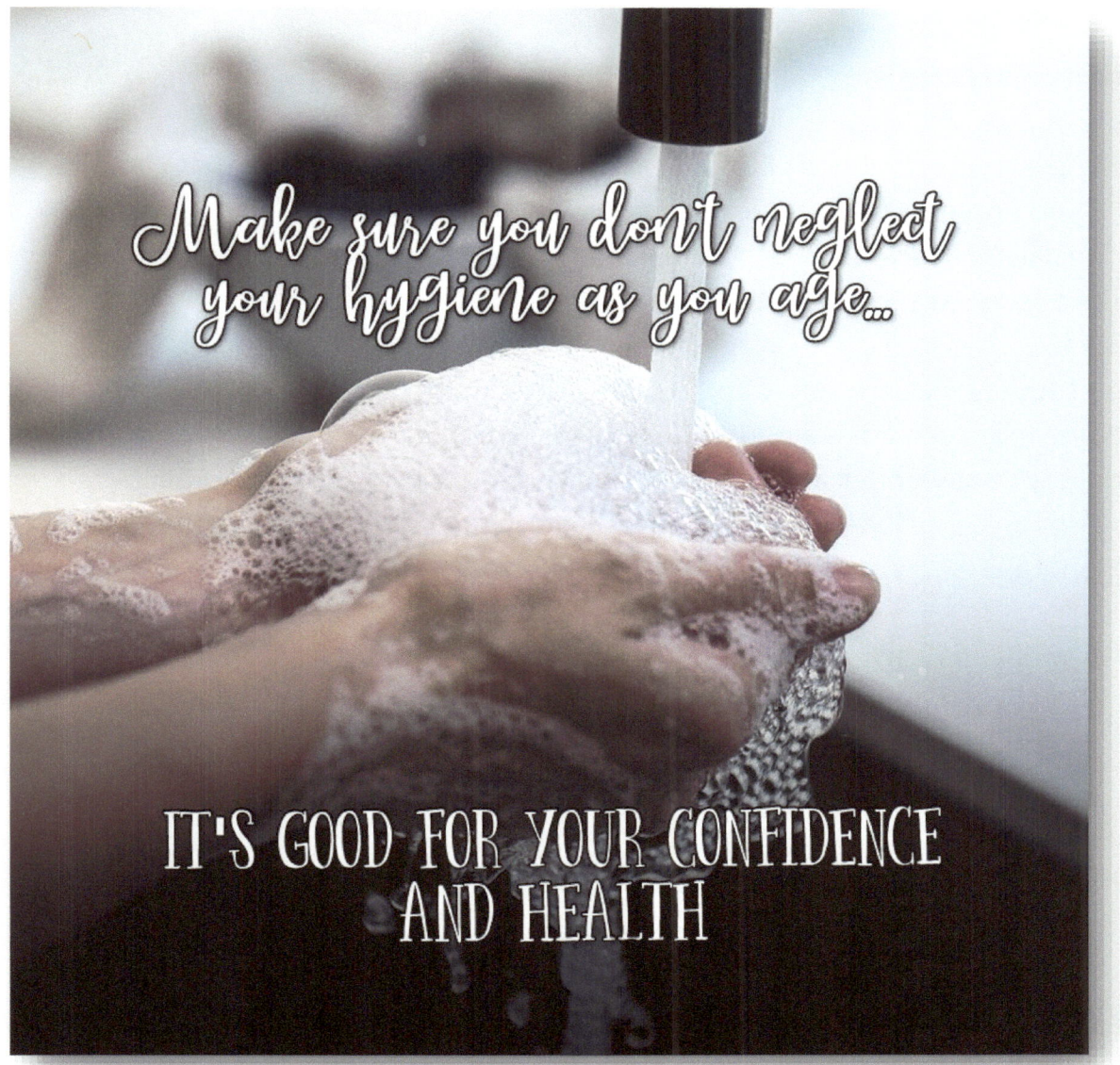

Do you feel proud and happy every time you hear a compliment? Of course, you do! If you're told you look fabulous, congratulate yourself on your obvious self-care.

Taking care of yourself with proper hygiene and grooming can add to your confidence and self-esteem. To receive a compliment for your efforts is inspiring.

Alternatively, poor personal hygiene can affect a person's social life and health. If you or someone you know needs a few helpful hygiene and grooming tips, we're here to help with a few suggestions below.

Bathing and Hair Care

Bathing is important. We all know that. It helps remove bacteria that causes body odor and prevents bacteria from growing and spreading on the body. It also washes away dead skin cells. Bathing also helps prevent the spread of infectious diseases such as the flu or common cold.

Use products that are suited for delicate, dry skin because your skin does tend to become more sensitive and dry as you age. Thoroughly clean all areas of the body, especially under any skin folds, which are prone to harboring bacteria. Problem areas include under the breasts, in the neck, in the stomach area, and the genitalia.

Rinse well and pat dry (don't rub) using an ultra-absorbent, soft bath towel to avoid chafing. Apply body lotion or moisturizer to keep the skin smooth, and wear a deodorant to keep you smelling fresh throughout the day.

Some deodorants can cause irritation and chafing due to their ingredients. If this is affecting you, look for products that do not contain aluminum, as it is the worst offender.

Wash your hair using a mild shampoo. Make sure you keep your scalp clean and give it a good massage when you do wash your hair or scalp. If your hair is excessively dry, you can use some oil treatments to protect your hair and scalp.

Hand Washing and Nails

Hand washing is and always has been, a major part of proper hygiene and sanitation, which helps decrease the risk of catching or spreading viral organisms. Using soap and water is still the best way to clean your hands.

Lather and rub your hands together for 20 seconds, and make sure you clean under your nails. Rinse well under warm running water and dry your hands.

Manicure your nails regularly, and if required, book yourself in for a pedicure. Don't let your toenails get forgotten! If you do not care for your feet, walking can and will become difficult. Don't be embarrassed about getting help, as foot care can become very difficult as mobility declines.

Oral Hygiene

As you age, your bones weaken, and so do your teeth. Your gums are also prone to developing periodontal disease caused by the bacteria in the plaque. This can make your gums swollen and they can bleed. Your breath won't smell very nice either if you have poor oral hygiene.

There are several things you can do to maintain good oral health. Brush at least twice a day, or if possible, after every meal. Your toothbrush should be 'soft' and replaced every three months at least. Floss every day to remove any plaque left behind from brushing. It is good to floss before brushing so that all debris is washed away. Rinse with mouthwash to remove any remaining bacteria.

If you wear dentures, make sure to follow your dentist's instructions for cleaning and maintenance. Visit your dentist regularly or as needed, to make sure you have no serious gum or mouth problems.

Skin

Your skin is the biggest organ of your body, so take special care of it. Use sunblock to protect your skin if necessary; however, make sure you aren't blocking out all the sun's rays as you need vitamin D. Use cleansers and moisturizers that suit your skin type.

If you are not capable of performing any of these routine tasks on your own, hire the help of a caregiver or specialist. Also, inquire as to any aged care service groups that may be able to assist you. Your hygiene and grooming are important to your physical and emotional health, so don't neglect yourself!

Conclusion

No-one really wants to grow old. Most people accept it, but some deeply struggle with the loss of the faculties they had when younger.

Acceptance of the inevitability of aging, and even 'growing older gracefully' doesn't mean blithely accepting that we have to become useless shadows of our former selves.

The great truth, as repeated often in this document, is that the so-called effects of aging have more to do with our actions and lifestyles than the passing of the years.

It is too easy, unfortunately, to take the easy path. To avoid discomfort, we exercise less. To save us having to deal with others, we avoid socializing. We eat comfort foods, and prepacked, processed foods, because it is easier.

This causes a downward spiral – we move less and actively think less. We move in smaller and smaller circles until we all but stop, and then we do.

However, we have the ability, in most cases, to take positive action that can reduce and reverse these diminishing effects. We can become more powerful and dynamic, and remain so for longer.

Follow the guidance given and live a more vibrant and joyous life, for as long as you can!

Recommended Resources

In the book there are several words that are highlighted. Below are those words and the correspondings to these recommended resources that can give you more information on that topic.

The links ending in numbers are hardcopy printed books that will be sent to you in the mail when purchased.

Links ending in a combination of letters and numbers are in digital Kindle format and will be moved to your Amazon online library after purchasing where you can download them to your e-reader device.

- Balance - https://www.amazon.com/gp/product/1530225779

- Daily Tasks - https://www.amazon.com/gp/product/B07FK5Q77R

- Vitamin D - https://www.amazon.com/gp/product/B075W3NBLQ

- Sitting - https://www.amazon.com/Reasons-Why-Sitting-Much-Kill-ebook/dp/B078GR5CJ8

- Heart-healthy habits - https://www.amazon.com/gp/product/B00WRCHCRS

- Stretches - https://www.amazon.com/gp/product/1980559562

About the Author

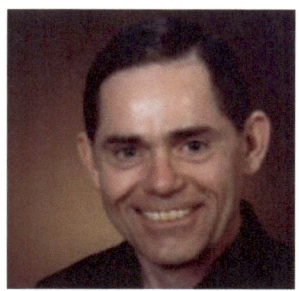

I have published numerous books on Amazon for Kindle and other publishing platforms. Both in electronic and POD formats.

While most of my books are on health and fitness in general, my topics of interest are leaning more toward aging baby boomers and the older population, such as is the topic of this book.

Besides my own writing, I also ghostwrite ebooks, books, reports, articles, blogs and do Kindle conversions for clients on a variety of topics. Go to my website at http://ronknesswriting.com for more information or to submit a quote. For a complete list of my books, go to https://www.amazon.com/Ron-Kness/e/B0072M6PYO.

Today my wife and I are retired from our careers and live in San Tan Valley, AZ. I now write as a retirement business where you'll find me happily sitting in my office typing away on my laptop as I work on my next book or ghostwriting project . . . that is if we are not traveling on a cruise ship - our new-found mode of travel.